I0416327

Diet, Exercise, and Sleep Trump
Medications
Medication is the Last Option
Your Fourth Psychiatric Consultation
Copyright Applied for 12/15/2019
all rights reserved.
William R. Yee M.D., J.D.

Healthy living habits start in childhood.

"Moderation in All Things," along with
the, "Golden Rule," treat others the way
you wish to be treated are thoughts that
permeate religions, philosophy, and
science.

Moderation promotes physical,
intellectual and emotional health which
make for more effective social, academic
and recreational efforts.

A life of moderation will do more for your
physical and mental health than all the
pills I can prescribe for you during your
lifetime.

The bell-shaped curve describes
moderation and extremes in physiologic
functions.

One standard deviation encompasses 68% of the population. Two standard deviations encompass 95% of the population.

How does one use standard deviations to describe moderation?

The Bell-Shaped Curve describes distribution of an attribute among the general population.

The notion of moderation must be individualized. Moderation may be described as the zone of maximum value such as optimum blood pressure, optimum quality of life, or longest life span.

Stimulation is one of the most critical variables that is addressed by psychiatrists.

Stimulation is measured along a continuum of low to high stimulation. Low stimulation is experienced as boredom.
Increase the stimulation and you experience pleasure. Increase the stimulation further and you experience stress.

The figure below is a rough example of what a Bell Shape Curve looks like with one standard deviation above and below the average enclosing 68% of the population and two standard deviations above and below the mean enclosing 95% of the population.

There is an optimum amount of stimulation for physical and mental health.
That optimum is different for each individual. Each individual should explore the boundaries of stimulation to determine what is boring, what is pleasure and what is painful. The figure below describes insufficient stimulation as boring and too much stimulation as panic.

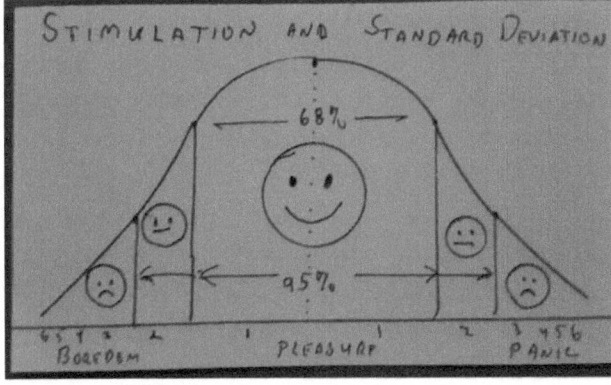

Some people experience excess
stimulation as a thrill instead of as a
panic. They seek thrills.
It is a matter of point of view and
attitude.

Some experience low levels of stimulation
as peacefulness instead of boredom.
It is a matter of point of view and
attitude.

Attitude determines whether a thrill or
panic is experienced. Panic, rage, and
thrill are all the product of high levels of
adrenalin which increases blood pressure
and heart rate which is experienced as
panic, thrill, or rage.

This book focuses on exercise, sleep and
diet to maximize quality of life. There are
many other activities. As you engage in
those activities, you should explore the
boundaries of those activities. You should
determine how extensive and intensive
these activities should be to extract your
optimum quality of life.

Let us start with diet.

The first concept that should be considered is the LD50. The LD50 is the lethal dose which kills half of those exposed to that dose.

Consider water. The LD50 for water is six liters. Half of the adults who drink six liters of water rapidly will die.

Consider alcohol. Half of the people who rapidly drink thirteen shots of liquor will die. A shot is 45 milliliters of 40% by volume alcohol.

A teaspoon of caffeine has 3.2 grams of caffeine. About 10 grams or three teaspoons of pure caffeine is a lethal dose.

A moderate or optimal level of water for daily consumption is between eight and fifteen, eight-ounce cups of water for the average adult male and eight to eleven, eight-ounce cups of water for an adult female.

Two to four cups of coffee daily reduce depression and with a reduction of depression one would expect a reduction in suicide.

For the average person 70 to 500 milligrams of coffee in the morning reduces the risk of depression and suicide. One cup has 70–140 mg of caffeine.

"Coffee, Caffeine, and Risk of Depression Among Women," Michel Lucas, PhD, RD; Fariba Mirzaei, MD, MPH, ScD; An Pan, PhD; et alOlivia I. Okereke, MD, SM; Walter C. Willett, MD, DrPH; Éilis J. O'Reilly, ScD; Karestan Koenen, PhD; Alberto Ascherio, MD, DrPH; Arch Intern Med. 2011;171(17):1571-1578. doi:10.1001/archinternmed.2011.393

Fasting is a common practice for religiou and other reasons.

There is some evidence that fasting can improve metabolic health and may facilitate weight loss. The issue of fasting merits more research.

Fasting in moderation, like exercise in moderation, is likely to improve quality o life and health.

"Intermittent Fasting and Human Metabolic Health."
Ruth E. Patterson, PhD,1,2 Gail A. Laughlin, PhD,1,2 Dorothy D. Sears, PhD,1,3 Andrea Z. LaCroix, PhD,1,2 Catherine Marinac, BA,1,4 Linda C. Gallo, PhD,5 Sheri J. Hartman, PhD,1,2 Loki Natarajan, PhD,1,2 Carolyn M. Senger, MD,1,2 María Elena Martínez, PhD,1,2 and Adriana Villaseñor, PhD1,2
J Acad Nutr Diet. Author manuscript; available in PMC 2016 Aug 1.
Published in final edited form as:
J Acad Nutr Diet. 2015 Aug; 115(8): 1203–1212.
Published online 2015 Apr 6.
doi: 10.1016/j.jand.2015.02.018
PMCID: PMC4516560
NIHMSID: NIHMS663671
PMID: 25857868

"Coffee and caffeine consumption and depression: A meta-analysis of observational studies."
Wang L, Shen X, Wu Y, Zhang D.
Aust N Z J Psychiatry. 2016 Mar;50(3):228-42. doi: 10.1177/0004867415603131. Epub 2015 Sep 2.

Maintaining healthy eating with a body mass index between 19 and 25 will lengthen life and reduce the risk of healt problems.

A healthy BMI for men and women is between 19 and 25. Consult with your doctor.

Approximate healthy weights for BMI of 19-25

Height — Weight
4'10" —— 91 to 115 pounds
4'11" —— 94 to 119 pounds
5'00" —— 97 to 123 pounds
5'01" —— 100 to 127 pounds
5'02" —— 104 to 131 pounds
5'03" —— 107 to 135 pounds
5'04" —— 110 to 140 pounds
5'05" —— 114 to 144 pounds
5'06" —— 118 to 148 pounds
5'07" —— 121 to 153 pounds
5'08" —— 125 to 158 pounds
5'09" —— 128 to 162 pounds
5'10" —— 132 to 167 pounds
5'11" —— 136 to 172 pounds
6'00" —— 140 to 177 pounds
6'01" —— 144 to 182 pounds
6'02" —— 148 to 186 pounds
6'03" —— 152 to 192 pounds

6'04" —— 156 to 205 pounds
6'05" —— 162 to 211 pounds
6'06" —— 164 to 216 pounds
6'07" —— 169 to 222 pounds
6'08" —— 173 to 228 pounds
6'09" —— 177 to 233 pounds
6'10" —— 182 to 239 pounds

Let us start with the adverse effects of
obesity.
As the BMI rises from 25 to 50 many
health problems emerge. The health
problems of obesity defeat medications
and surgical treatments for obesity.

Obesity increases fat in the belly, liver,
heart, brain, prostate gland, arteries, skin
and other organs.

Let's start with the brain. Fat in the brain
causes the brain to expand.
Unfortunately, the brain is in the skull
which protects the brain from damage
due to blunt trauma such as falls.

When the brain expands it puts pressure
on the brain stem and optic nerves which
are near openings that relieve pressure
on the brain.

The result on the optic nerve is pseudo tumor cerebri. The fat puts pressure on the optic nerve and acts like a false tumor.

Intracranial hypertension from obesity has been reported commonly and can even affect children and adolescents.

Headaches with obesity are a warning sign of intracranial hypertension and pseudotumor cerebri.

When the doctor looks into the eye at the optic nerve, he sees that pseudotumor cerebri causes swelling of the optic nerve which can lead to loss of vision.

Pseudotumor cerebri headaches sometimes manifests as pain behind the eyes.

Sometimes the patient can hear the blood pulsing in the arteries of the head with pseudotumor cerebri.

Intracranial pressure can result in nause and vomiting that can also occur with subdural hematomas from head injuries.

There may be loss of visual acuity, (loss of the ability to perceive fine details), or loss of portions of the visual fields with pseudotumor cerebri. The most common visual field defect is increase in the blind spot size. The second most common visual defect is loss of portions of the medial or nasal sides of the visual fields in both eyes. The loss of visual acuity and visual fields is associated with chronic papilledema, or chronic swelling of the optic nerve.

Simply said, the longer the patient has swelling of the brain and swelling of the optic nerve, the more likely there will be permanent loss of visual fields and visual acuity.

Respiratory problems are common with obesity and increase in severity with the severity of the obesity.
Accumulation of fat in the chest and abdomen results in mechanical compression of the diaphragm. This does not allow the diaphragm to move. The diaphragm allows for breathing when asleep because the brain stem drives the diaphragm while you sleep.

With the diaphragm paralyzed by fat, breathing stops with sleep and the sleeper awakens. This is Ondine's Curse, a paralyzed diaphragm, and a life without sleep.

Fat accumulates in the liver resulting in an enlarged and fatty liver. This is called Non-Alcoholic Fatty Liver Disease, NAFLD and, is accompanied by Steatosis, accumulation of fat in the liver, with or without fibrosis, steatohepatitis. The medical literature reports death from liver failure and renal failure due to obesity.

Obesity stresses the kidneys directly due to the direct metabolic stress on the kidneys created by obesity. In addition, obesity increases hypertension and diabetes which also injure the kidneys. Obesity increases chronic kidney disease and death from kidney failure.

Obesity increases coronary heart disease and death from heart attacks and heart failure.
Obesity increases the risk of stroke and all the complications of stroke including death.

Diet, exercise and weight loss can reverse all the above side effects and risks of obesity.

By-pass surgery for obesity has severe life-threatening side effects and a high failure rate.

Obesity affects the prostate gland and causes both Benign Prostatic Hypertrophy with urinary obstruction and Prostate Cancer according to literature easily found on the internet.

There is no organ in the body that is spared due to the direct effects of fat accumulation and the indirect effects of diabetes and cardiovascular disease,

Medical interventions for obesity are not very effective and as a result a variety of gastric surgeries have emerged as a last resort for obesity. They have serious side effects and a rather high failure rate.

The Gold Standard for obesity is eighty to ninety percent eat less and ten to twenty percent exercise more.

The only effective intervention for obesity is to eat less and be hungry. There is no way to lose weight except to eat less.

There is no way to eat less without being hungry. If you are not losing weight you are not hungry enough and you are eating too much.

No excuses, no explanations, nature cannot be defeated. You cannot lie to nature.

You can lie to your spouse, your children your employer, your insurance company and your doctor. You cannot lie to the weight scales.
Either you are losing weight, or you are eating too much,

I have never had a morbidly obese patient with diabetes, hypertension, headaches, impaired vision, a fatty liver, chronic renal disease, with difficulty breathing tell me they were happy.

I have not been successful in treating obesity and refer obese patients to eating disorders clinics as I do not have the tool to resolve obesity.

What does the medical literature tell us about the treatment of obesity? Good question.

Obesity is associated with Binge Eating, Bulimia, Anorexia Nervosa and a host of medical problems starting with early onset Diabetes Mellites with all the complications that go with diabetes.

Obesity and anorexia are in the posture that male erectile dysfunction was before the discovery of Viagra. No simple and effective treatment exists.

Obesity and anorexia are poorly understood neurophysiological dysfunctions.
When the neurophysiological dysfunctions are understood there will be a, "Viagra-neurophysiological-obesity pill," and a "Viagra-neurophysiological-anorexia pill," that will resolve obesity and anorexia as efficiently as Viagra resolves male impotence.

Recent review of the medical literature reveals that treatment of obesity is not very effective and the long-term impact of interventions are not known.

"Overview of meta-analysis on prevention and treatment of childhood obesity."

Bahia L1, Schaan CW2, Sparrenberger K3 Abreu GA4, Barufaldi LA5, Coutinho W6, Schaan BD7.

J Pediatr (Rio J). 2019 Jul - Aug;95(4):385-400. doi: 10.1016/j.jped.2018.07.009. Epub 2018 Aug 16.

Most studies on obesity are short term, and there is no single intervention that has been able to prevent surgery.

Surgery for morbid obesity is effective. However, effective is not a cure. Effective is a partial and uncertain reduction in weight. Surgery sometimes needs to be repeated and surgical complications are substantial and include death.

"The effectiveness and risks of bariatric surgery: an updated systematic review and meta-analysis," 2003-2012.

Chang SH1, Stoll CR1, Song J2, Varela JE3, Eagon CJ3, Colditz GA1.

JAMA Surg. 2014 Mar;149(3):275-87. doi: 10.1001/jamasurg.2013.3654.

In summary, you are better off if you control your dietary intake.

Learn to fast in moderation.

Learn to stop eating when you are still hungry to lose weight.

If you are underweight, learn to eat when you are not hungry.

Eat the calories you require to achieve and maintain your ideal weight.

The hardest lessen in life is learning to control your appetites and your impulses.

Master yourself and you master the art of living.

After eating, sleeping is the next life activity with common issues that result in a doctor's appointment.

Most normal people experience insomnia for a day or more depending upon circumstances.

Twenty five percent of people have insomnia every year and three out of four recover and one out of four suffer an extended period of insomnia.

Chronic insomnia is reported to range from three to thirty three percent of population samples. The patient populations sampled vary as does the definition of insomnia.

Associations that treat insomnia tend to report a higher rate of insomnia than groups that do not treat insomnia.

Babies are born without ninety-minute REM cycles that are the basis of normal sleep in adults.

Babies have fifty-minute REM cycles that mature to ninety-minute REM cycles in their ninth month on average.

Maturation of physiologic functions have a wide range on the calendar.

Physiologic functions are not tied directl to the calendar and are affected by a wid variety of intervening variables including diet, weather, family, DNA, community, and cultural environments.

It is believed that REM sleep is a time during which the brain processes the daily experiences into memories and consolidates the daily learning with lifetime experiences.

The details are not completely known. It is known that memories are reconstructed and generally not recalled with digital accuracy.

Memories are generally analogue representations of a single event through the lens of a life of learning.

Insomnia is defined as lack of normal sleep.

Physiologic functions fall on a spectrum of extremes from the rare complete absence to the rare complete presence.

For insomnia there would be the complete absence due to Ondine's curse to the complete presence due to a coma from a head injury.

Ondine's Curse is due to damage anywhere from the respiratory center located in the medulla oblongata to paralysis of the phrenic nerve to the diaphragm.

Ondine's Curse occurs if the person stops breathing when he falls into asleep. When the breathing stops the person wakes up. The result is a life without sleep.

Adults with Guillain Barre post viral polyneuropathy can stop breathing due to damage to this same neurological array from the brain to the diaphragm.

The respiratory arrest wakes the patient up.

It is necessary to put the patient into an iron lung to breathe for the patient or have some other mechanical respiration when he wants to sleep.

Tracheotomy and ventilators have the drawback of infections and other complications.

Iron lungs were used to keep polio patients alive when they couldn't breathe because of damage to the neurological array between the brain and diaphragm.

Sleep apnea from mechanical pressure.

Fat in the liver and abdomen creates mechanical pressure on the diaphragm that can cause sleep apnea, respiratory arrest and insomnia.

Pickwickian Syndrome is an early description of respiratory problems from fat in the abdomen paralyzing the diaphragm.

Acid reflux can cause insomnia due to irritation of the vocal cords and respiratory distress.

Restless legs and other movement disorders during sleep can cause insomnia.

Malfunction of the sleep cycle due to neurophysiologic impairments, medical problems, medications, sleep apnea and street drugs can cause insomnia.

Insomnia can be due to an abnormal circadian rhythm that can be shorter than 24 hours, longer than 24 hours or otherwise pathological.

Abnormal behavior patterns can lead to insomnia from mental illness or bad habits.

Shift work and poor sleep hygiene can cause insomnia. Work in foundries, emergency rooms and other environment often require that the employee rotate through the first, second and third shift every ninety days or so. The rotation can be retrograde or anterograde.

If the employee is required to move to a later shift and stay up longer the transition to normal sleep is easier than i the employee is required to go to an earlier shift and start sleeping earlier. It is easier to sleep later than earlier than the normal bedtime.

This leads to the topic of sleep hygiene.

Sleep hygiene is a pattern of behavior that promotes or disrupts healthy sleep.

For optimum sleep a person should get u and go to bed at the same time every day.

In general, it is best to get up with the su rise and go to sleep after dark.

Eight to ten hours of sleep on average is optimum for good physical and mental health.

The bell-shaped curve for healthy sleep is in fact six to ten hours of sleep for the general population.

Healthy sleep is different for each person. Each person has a normal range of sleep that varies from night to night.

It is necessary to keep a sleep diary to determine what a person's normal sleep is for optimum physical and mental health.

It is necessary to keep a sleep diary to determine what is the normal variation in hours of sleep per night for each individual.

The sleep diary should record the number and time of beverages with caffeine.

The sleep diary should include the time and amount of physical activity and meals.

The sleep diary should include the time and amount of medications taken.

The sleep diary should include the type of work and duration for each day.

The sleep diary should include the types and severity of daily stressors and the types and significance of positive social, educational, vocational, and health events.

The sleep diary should include the duration and quality of sleep and the energy and fatigue levels upon arising, during the day and at bedtime.

There should be daily, weekly, and monthly reviews of the sleep diary.

The activities and experiences that improve sleep or cause insomnia should be tracked during the year and the effect of interventions to improve sleep should also be tracked.

Sleep hygiene generally requires going to sleep and getting up at the same time each morning.

Two or three cups of coffee in the morning has been associated with a reduction of depression and suicide.

Switching from caffeinated beverages in the morning to chamomile tea in the afternoon and evening is associated with improved sleep.

Taking melatonin in the evening is associated with improved sleep.

If sleep hygiene does not maintain healthy sleep, I recommend a sleep EEG and a consultation with a sleep clinic to sort out the different medical conditions and sleep disorders that impair sleep.

You could be suffering from Narcolepsy and a host of other medical problems with specific interventions that improve sleep.

I recommend against the long-term use of a sleeping pill.

Sleeping pills are addicting and lose their effect within fourteen days.

Insomnia is in the posture of male impotence before the discovery of Viagra. Lacking Viagra for Insomnia, it is necessary to have a sleep EEG and a consultation with a sleep clinic to properly diagnose and treat insomnia.

Zolpidem/Ambien and benzodiazepines are used for insomnia. They are addicting and I do not recommend them for long term use.

Other problems with Zolpidem/Ambien and benzodiazepines include confusion, falls and hip fractures in the elderly. In any age group there are dissociative states reported including sleep eating, sleep sex, sleep driving. Attorneys have used the "Ambien Defense," to acquit defendants from charges of homicide.

More than seventy percent of patients on Ambien continue Ambien after fourteen days although it is known to lose effect after fourteen days. I ask, "physicians prescribe medications, but patients ignore FDA safety recommendations?" What say you?

"77% of patients ignore FDA safety recommendations for Ambien"
Moore TJ, et al. JAMA Intern Med. 2018;doi:10.1001/jamainternmed.2018.303
July 19, 2018

I say that the literature supporting medication for insomnia is based upon short term studies that cannot address issues of addiction properly. What say you?

"Benzodiazepines and zolpidem for chronic insomnia: a meta-analysis of treatment efficacy."
Nowell PD1, Mazumdar S, Buysse DJ, Dew MA, Reynolds CF 3rd, Kupfer DJ.
JAMA. 1997 Dec 24-31;278(24):2170-7.

Cognitive Behavior Therapy seems to be the most effective treatment for insomnia.

Cognitive and behavioral therapies in the treatment of insomnia: A meta-analysis
Annemieke van Straten, Tanja van der Zweerde a, Annet Kleiboer a, Pim Cuijpers a, Charles M. Morin b , Jaap Lancee
Sleep Med Rev. 2018 Apr;38:3-16. doi: 10.1016/j.smrv.2017.02.001. Epub 2017 Feb 9.   PMID: 28392168
DOI: 10.1016/j.smrv.2017.02.001

Long term use of sleeping pills are generally contraindicated as the adverse effects of addiction and habituation outweigh the benefits which are generally short-term effectiveness that wanes and dissipates with habituation and addiction after the first two weeks.

"Behavioral and pharmacologic therapies for chronic insomnia in adults,"
<u>Michael H Bonnet, PhD</u>
<u>Donna L Arand, PhD</u>
Section Editor:
<u>Ruth Benca, MD, PhD</u>
Deputy Editor:
<u>April F Eichler, MD, MPH</u>

In summary, moderation in all things supports a healthy sleep pattern.

Going to bed and getting up the same time every day is very important for high quality sleep, physical and mental health.

Personal discipline in these matters is part of the lifelong task of mastering yourself. You can do it.

Now we address the topic of exercise.

Daily exercise reduces anxiety, reduces depression and improves sleep.
Exercise should be started slowly with light exercise and should be increased slowly.

This allows the tendons and ligaments to increase in strength and prevent injuries.

Muscles tend to increase in strength faster than ligaments and tendons.

Aggressive exercise can lead to injuries to tendons and ligaments.

Start with low levels of exercise and increase exercise slowly. This cautious approach to exercise prevents injury and allows for integration of exercise into the daily routine with minimal disruption of other life activities.

One pound, two pound, three pound, four pound, five pound, six pound, seven pound, eight pound, nine pound and ten pound dumbbell sets are inexpensive.

These dumb bells allow for start low and go slow routines at home. Generally, an exercise routine at home can be done in the time that it takes to travel to the gym.

The exercise routine can be done in the morning before work with a few cups of coffee.

Daily exercise as a lifelong routine is the most effective strategy for moderation and for good physical and mental health.

Exercise is effective for reducing depression and anxiety.

"Effects of exercise on depression and anxiety in persons living with HIV: A meta-analysis,"
Heissel A1, Zech P2, Rapp MA2, Schuch FB3, Lawrence JB2, Kangas M4, Heinzel S5.
J Psychosom Res. 2019 Nov;126:109823. doi: 10.1016/j.jpsychores.2019.109823. Epu 2019 Sep 2.

The literature that describes a small effect for medications on depression and anxiety implies the fact that exercise may be as effective as medications for depression and anxiety.

Analysis of the research concludes that the research is of poor quality and medications are not much more effective than placebo for depression for mild, moderate and severe depression.

"Initial severity of major depression and efficacy of new generation antidepressants: individual participant data meta-analysis."
Furukawa TA, Maruo K, Noma H, Tanaka S, Imai H, Shinohara K, Ikeda K, Yamawaki S, Levine SZ, Goldberg Y, Leucht S, Cipriani A.
Acta Psychiatr Scand. 2018 Jun;137(6):450-458. doi: 10.1111/acps.12886. Epub 2018 Apr 3.

"Efficacy and Safety of Selective Serotonin Reuptake Inhibitors, Serotonin-Norepinephrine Reuptake Inhibitors, and Placebo for Common Psychiatric Disorders Among Children and Adolescents A Systematic Review and Meta-analysis,"
Cosima Locher, PhD1;
Helen Koechlin, MSc; Sean R. Zion, MA; et al Christoph Werner, BSc; Daniel S. Pine, MD; Irving Kirsch, PhD; Ronald C. Kessler, PhD; Joe Kossowsky, PhD, MMSc
JAMA Psychiatry. 2017;74(10):1011-1020. doi:10.1001/jamapsychiatry.2017.2432

If you have medical conditions such as heart conditions, skeletal malformations, and other medical conditions you should consult with a cardiologist, orthopedic surgeon, or physiatrist for a recommendation regarding exercise and possibly work with a physical therapist t learn how to exercise correctly to avoid physical injury.

In general, swimming is the best exercise because it takes the weight off joints while allowing for a good cardiovascular workout.

In general, aerobic exercise that increase the heart rate is superior to non-aerobic exercise.

Moderation in all things, mastering yourself, and daily small changes lead to the optimum life style and best quality of life.

Religion can be seen through the lens of history as science before the scientific method.

Religious clerics in the middle ages brought Greek philosophy and math and science back to life and started the renaissance of science in the western culture.

"The Golden Rule," is a bridge between science and religion. The golden rule is a basic tenet in most religions. "The Golden Rule," is implied in Sun Tzu's book, <u>The Art of War.</u> Sun Tzu stated that war was a failure of politics. This also implied moderation as war is an extreme measure.

"The Golden Rule," is a part of a winning strategy in the science of game theory. Game theory is the science of conflict as manifested in politics, war, and sports.

The point of discussing the, "Golden Rule," here is that it is an important part of moderation in all things. Making friends instead of enemies is part of moderation in all things. In general, it is better to give a little more than you receive.

Casting bread upon the waters embraces the idea that it comes back sevenfold.

Charity and hospitality are investments in the community with intangible as well as tangible rewards.

A community with charity and hospitality is a stable, low conflict community that fosters good mental health.

Moderation in all things includes pursuing a variety of interests and activities.

Variety is the spice of life.

Variety is an antidote to boredom.

Zen Buddhism embraces beauty in simplicity. Simplicity allows for low energy meditation and peace of mind that balances the complexity and stimulation created by contests in sports and politics.

A balance of simplicity and complexity, a balance of peace and stress, balance among all dimensions is a means of achieving moderation in all things while exploring boundaries and variety.

Moderation in sleep, eating and exercise all contribute to good health.
Exploring boundaries and your tolerance to boredom and stress as you approach boundaries is part of learning to master your interests, appetites and addictions.

Wisdom and peace of mind can be yours.

Mastery of your interests, appetites and addictions is mastery of life.

Mastery of your interests and addictions is a means of acquiring wisdom and peace of mind as you mature into late life.

Wisdom and peace of mind embrace all that is important in life.

Thank you for your time and attention.

William R. Yee M.D., J.D.   12/15/2019
Board Certified Psychiatrist

"Pre-Existing text," includes names of Symptoms and medical illnesses, medications, people, corporations, law cases, statutes, text of statutes, the titles of articles and books, the content of articles and books cited.

My copyright claim is a claim to the "original text," which is my personal experiences as described in the text above and my commentary on the names of symptoms and medical illnesses, medications, people, corporations, law cases, statutes, text of statutes, the titles of articles and books, the content of articles and books cited.

www.ingramcontent.com/pod-product-compliance
Lightning Source LLC
Chambersburg PA
CBHW050353290526
45785CB00006B/2749